Herbal

Remedies and Recipes

for Kings

A Guide to Optimal Health

By Nicole Archa

Table Of Contents

Dedicated To My Brothers

Introduction

Herbal remedies have been used for centuries to treat various ailments in men. These remedies are made from natural plants, herbs, and other botanicals that have medicinal properties. Herbal remedies are considered to be a safe and effective alternative to traditional medications, as they have fewer side effects and are less likely to interact with other medications.

One of the most popular herbal remedies for men is Saw Palmetto. This herb is commonly used to treat symptoms of an enlarged prostate, also known as benign prostatic hyperplasia (BPH). Saw Palmetto works by blocking the conversion of testosterone to dihydrotestosterone (DHT), which is a hormone that can cause the prostate to enlarge. This herb can also be used to improve urinary symptoms and sexual function in men.

Another popular herbal remedy for men is Ginkgo Biloba. This herb has been used for thousands of years in traditional Chinese medicine and has been found to improve blood flow, particularly to the brain and the legs. Ginkgo Biloba can be used to improve sexual function and to treat symptoms of erectile dysfunction. It may also help with memory problems, depression, and anxiety.

Tribulus Terrestris is an herb that has been used to treat sexual dysfunction and improve athletic performance. This herb works by increasing the level of testosterone in the body, which can help with sexual function, muscle growth, and energy levels. It may also help with infertility and low sperm count.

Ashwagandha is an herb that is commonly used in Ayurvedic medicine to help the body cope with stress and anxiety. It is also used to improve sexual function and fertility in men. Ashwagandha works by reducing the levels of cortisol, a hormone that is associated with stress, and increasing the levels of testosterone.

Another popular herbal remedy for men is Horny Goat Weed. This herb has been used for centuries in traditional Chinese medicine to improve sexual function and libido. It works by increasing the levels of nitric oxide in the body, which can help with blood flow and sexual function.

Other herbal remedies for men include Maca Root, which is used to improve energy and sexual function, and Epimedium, which is used to improve sexual function and libido.

It is important to note that before taking any herbal remedy, it is important to speak with a healthcare professional, as some herbs can interact with other medications or have side effects. It is also important to ensure that the herbs are obtained from a reputable source and are of high quality.

In conclusion, herbal remedies can be an effective and safe alternative to traditional medications for men. Some of the most popular herbal remedies for men include Saw Palmetto, Ginkgo Biloba, Tribulus Terrestris, Ashwagandha, Horny Goat Weed, Maca Root and Epimedium. These herbs can be used to treat symptoms of an enlarged prostate, improve sexual function, increase energy levels, and reduce stress and anxiety. However, it is important to consult a healthcare professional before taking any herbal remedy, and to ensure that the herbs are obtained from a reputable source.

Overview of herbal remedies for men's health

Herbal remedies have been used for centuries to treat various ailments in men's health. These remedies are made from natural plants, herbs, and other botanicals that have medicinal properties. Herbal remedies are considered to be a safe and effective alternative to traditional medications, as they have fewer side effects and are less likely to interact with other medications.

One of the most popular herbal remedies for men's health is Saw Palmetto. This herb is commonly used to treat symptoms of an enlarged prostate, also known as benign prostatic hyperplasia (BPH). Saw Palmetto works by blocking the conversion of testosterone to dihydrotestosterone (DHT), which is a hormone that can cause the prostate to enlarge. This herb can also be used to improve urinary symptoms and sexual function in men.

Another popular herbal remedy for men's health is Ginkgo Biloba. This herb has been used for thousands of years in traditional Chinese medicine and has been found to improve blood flow, particularly to the brain and the legs. Ginkgo Biloba can be used to improve sexual function and to treat symptoms of erectile dysfunction. It may also help with memory problems, depression, and anxiety.

Tribulus Terrestris is an herb that has been used to treat sexual dysfunction and improve athletic performance. This herb works by increasing the level of testosterone in the body, which can help with sexual function, muscle growth, and energy levels. It may also help with infertility and low sperm count.

Ashwagandha is an herb that is commonly used in Ayurvedic medicine to help the body cope with stress and anxiety. It is also used to improve sexual function and fertility in men. Ashwagandha works by reducing the levels of cortisol, a hormone that is associated with stress, and increasing the levels of testosterone.

Another popular herbal remedy for men's health is Horny Goat Weed. This herb has been used for centuries in traditional Chinese medicine to improve sexual function and libido. It works by increasing the levels of nitric oxide in the body, which can help with blood flow and sexual function.

Other herbal remedies for men's health include Maca Root, which is used to improve energy and sexual function, and Epimedium, which is used to improve sexual function and libido.

Herbal remedies can also be used to treat other men's health issues such as prostate cancer, hair loss, and male pattern baldness. Saw

Palmetto, for example, has been found to have anti-cancer properties and may be useful in the treatment of prostate cancer. Saw Palmetto is also believed to be beneficial for preventing hair loss and promoting hair growth.

Herbal remedies can also be used to treat other men's health issues such as prostate cancer, hair loss, and male pattern baldness. Saw Palmetto, for example, has been found to have anti-cancer properties and may be useful in the treatment of prostate cancer. Saw Palmetto is also believed to be beneficial for preventing hair loss and promoting hair growth.

Herbal remedies can also be used to improve overall health and wellness in men. For example, herbs such as Panax Ginseng and Cordyceps Sinensis have been found to improve energy levels, boost immunity and improve overall cardiovascular health.

Herbs like Turmeric and ginger are widely used for their anti-inflammatory properties and can be helpful in treating conditions such as osteoarthritis and rheumatoid arthritis. They can also be used to reduce pain and inflammation associated with injuries and surgeries.

Herbs like Milk Thistle and Dandelion are known for their liver-protective properties and can be used to improve liver function and detoxify the body.

Herbal remedies can also be used to improve mental health and cognitive function in men. For example, herbs like Bacopa Monnieri and Ginkgo Biloba have been found to improve memory and cognitive function. Similarly, herbs like St. John's Wort and Passionflower can be used to reduce symptoms of anxiety and depression.

In conclusion, herbal remedies can be an effective and safe alternative to traditional medications for men's health. Herbs such as Saw Palmetto, Ginkgo Biloba, Tribulus Terrestris, Ashwagandha, Horny Goat Weed, Maca Root and Epimedium can be used to treat various health issues in men including prostate problems, sexual dysfunction, and anxiety. Other herbs like Panax Ginseng, Cordyceps Sinensis, Turmeric, ginger, Milk Thistle, Dandelion, Bacopa Monnieri, Ginkgo Biloba, St. John's Wort, and Passionflower are also useful for improving overall health and wellness in men. However, it is important to consult a healthcare professional before taking any herbal remedy, and to ensure that the herbs are obtained from a reputable source.

The benefits of using herbal remedies

Herbal remedies have been used for centuries to treat various ailments and promote overall health and wellness. These remedies are made from natural plants, herbs, and other botanicals that have medicinal properties. Herbal remedies are considered to be a safe and effective alternative to traditional medications, as they have fewer side effects and are less likely to interact with other medications.

One of the main benefits of using herbal remedies is that they are natural and therefore have fewer side effects than traditional medications. Many prescription and over-the-counter medications can have serious side effects, such as stomach upset, headache, and allergic reactions. Herbal remedies, on the other hand, are generally considered to be safe when used as directed.

Another benefit of using herbal remedies is that they can be used to treat a wide variety of conditions. Herbs such as Saw Palmetto, Ginkgo Biloba, Tribulus Terrestris, Ashwagandha, Horny Goat Weed, Maca Root and Epimedium can be used to treat various health issues in men including prostate problems, sexual dysfunction, and anxiety. Other herbs like Panax Ginseng, Cordyceps Sinensis, Turmeric, ginger, Milk Thistle, Dandelion, Bacopa Monnieri, Ginkgo Biloba, St. John's Wort, and Passionflower are also useful for improving overall health and wellness in men.

Herbal remedies can also be used in combination with other treatments to provide a more comprehensive approach to healthcare. For example, herbs can be used in conjunction with conventional medications to manage symptoms of a chronic condition, such as diabetes or high blood pressure. Additionally, some herbal remedies can be used as a preventative measure to boost overall health and immunity.

Herbal remedies are also more accessible and affordable than traditional medications. Herbs can be easily obtained from health food stores, online retailers, or even grown in a home garden. They are also typically less expensive than prescription medications.

Another benefit of using herbal remedies is that they can be used in a variety of forms, such as teas, tinctures, capsules, or topical creams. This allows for a greater degree of customization and flexibility in treatment, as different forms may be more effective for different individuals or conditions.

Herbs also have cultural and traditional significance and have been used in various cultures for centuries, which is an added advantage. They are also known to be biocompatible with the human body, which means that the body can easily recognize and use the nutrients present in herbs.

Furthermore, herbal remedies can provide a holistic approach to healthcare, as they not only address the physical symptoms of a condition, but also take into account the emotional and spiritual aspects of an individual. Many herbs have been found to promote relaxation and stress relief, which can improve overall well-being. Herbs like ashwagandha and passionflower can be used to reduce anxiety and promote a sense of calm.

Herbal remedies can also be used to boost overall health and prevent illness. For example, herbs like echinacea and goldenseal can be used to boost immunity and prevent colds and flu. Other herbs, like turmeric and ginger, have anti-inflammatory properties and can be used to prevent chronic diseases such as osteoarthritis and rheumatoid arthritis.

Herbal remedies also have the potential to be more sustainable than traditional medications. Many traditional medications are derived from synthetic chemicals and can have negative impacts on the environment. Herbs, on the other hand, can be grown and harvested in a sustainable manner and are biodegradable.

In summary, herbal remedies can provide a safe and effective alternative to traditional medications, with many benefits such as fewer side effects, the ability to treat a wide variety of conditions, a holistic approach to healthcare, prevention of illness, accessibility, affordability and sustainability. However, it is important to consult a healthcare professional before taking any herbal remedy, and to ensure that the herbs are obtained from a reputable source.

Common Men's Health Issues

There are a variety of men's health issues that can be treated or improved with the use of herbal remedies. Some of the most common men's health issues that herbs can help with include:

Prostate problems: One of the most common men's health issues is prostate problems, such as an enlarged prostate or prostate cancer. Herbs like Saw Palmetto have been found to be effective in treating symptoms of an enlarged prostate and may also have anti-cancer properties.

Sexual dysfunction: Herbs like Horny Goat Weed, Tribulus Terrestris and Ginkgo Biloba have been found to be effective in improving sexual function and treating symptoms of erectile dysfunction. These herbs work by increasing blood flow to the penis and boosting levels of testosterone.

Hair loss and male pattern baldness: Herbs like Saw Palmetto and Ginkgo Biloba have been found to be effective in preventing hair loss and promoting hair growth. Saw Palmetto works by blocking the conversion of testosterone to dihydrotestosterone (DHT), which can cause hair loss.

Stress and anxiety: Herbs like Ashwagandha and Passionflower have been found to be effective in reducing symptoms of stress and anxiety. Ashwagandha works by reducing the levels of cortisol, a hormone associated with stress, while Passion flower is known to have a calming effect on the nervous system.

Infertility: Herbs like Tribulus Terrestris and Maca Root have been found to be effective in improving fertility in men. Tribulus Terrestris works by increasing the level of testosterone in the body, which can help with sperm production, while Maca Root is believed to improve sperm count and motility.

Cardiovascular health: Herbs like Panax Ginseng and Cordyceps Sinensis have been found to be effective in improving cardiovascular health. These herbs work by improving circulation, reducing cholesterol levels and managing hypertension.

Liver health: Herbs like Milk Thistle and Dandelion have been found to be effective in improving liver function and detoxifying the body. They help in protecting the liver from toxins and other harmful compounds.

Cognitive function: Herbs like Bacopa Monnieri and Ginkgo Biloba have been found to be effective in improving memory and cognitive function. These herbs

Another common men's health issue that can be treated with herbal remedies is digestive issues such as constipation, diarrhea, and acid reflux. Herbs such as ginger, peppermint, and fennel can be used to improve digestion and relieve symptoms of digestive discomfort.

Ginger is a popular herb that has been used for centuries to treat digestive issues. It is known to have anti-inflammatory properties and can be used to relieve nausea, vomiting, and stomach cramps. It also has been found to be effective in relieving symptoms of acid reflux and heartburn.

Peppermint is another herb that is commonly used to treat digestive issues. It has been found to be effective in relieving symptoms of stomach cramps, bloating and gas. Peppermint oil is also known to have a relaxing effect on the muscles in the digestive tract, which can help to relieve constipation and diarrhea.

Fennel is an herb that is commonly used to improve digestion and relieve symptoms of bloating and gas. It has been found to be effective in relieving symptoms of indigestion and acid reflux. It also has antispasmodic properties which can help to relieve stomach cramps and spasms.

In addition, probiotics, the live microorganisms which are similar to the beneficial microorganisms found in the human gut, can be used to improve digestion and boost the immune system. Probiotics can be found in fermented foods such as yogurt, kefir, and sauerkraut, and are also available in supplement form.

In conclusion, herbal remedies can be an effective and safe alternative to traditional medications for men's health. Herbs such as ginger, peppermint, fennel and probiotics can be used to treat various digestive issues in men including constipation, diarrhea, acid reflux, bloating, and gas. These herbs can improve digestion and boost the immune system. However, it is important to consult a healthcare professional before taking any herbal remedy, and to ensure that the herbs are obtained from a reputable source.

Herbs for erectile dysfunction

Erectile dysfunction (ED) is a common condition that affects many men, and it can be caused by a variety of factors such as age, diabetes, high blood pressure, and cardiovascular disease. ED is characterized by the inability to achieve or maintain an erection sufficient for sexual intercourse. While there are several medications available to treat ED, some men may prefer to try herbal remedies instead.

Ginkgo biloba is a popular herb that has been traditionally used to treat ED. Ginkgo is a natural antioxidant that helps improve blood flow to the genitals, which may help with ED. Studies have shown that ginkgo can improve sexual function in men with mild to moderate ED. However, it's important to note that more research is needed to confirm these findings.

Another popular herb for ED is horny goat weed. Horny goat weed is also believed to improve blood flow to the genitals, which can help with ED. It is also thought to help with other sexual problems such as premature ejaculation and low libido. Some studies have found that horny goat weed may improve sexual function in men with ED, but more research is needed to confirm these findings.

Panax ginseng is another herb that has been traditionally used to treat ED. Panax ginseng is believed to improve overall sexual function, including ED. Studies have found that panax ginseng can improve sexual function in men with ED, but more research is needed to confirm these findings.

Yohimbe is an herb that is derived from the bark of a tree native to West Africa, and it is believed to help with ED by improving blood flow to the genitals. Yohimbe is available in supplement form, but it can also be found in some over-the-counter male enhancement products. Studies have found that yohimbe can help improve ED in some men, but it can also cause side effects such as high blood pressure, anxiety, and headaches. Therefore, it is important to talk to a healthcare professional before using yohimbe.

DHEA, Dehydroepiandrosterone is another natural hormone that's been used to improve sexual function, and it's been found to be effective in some men with ED. DHEA is a natural hormone that's made by the adrenal glands. The body converts DHEA into testosterone and estrogen. Some studies have found that DHEA can improve sexual function in men with ED, but more research is needed to confirm these findings.

It's important to note that while these herbs may be effective, they can also have side effects and may interact with other medications you are taking. Therefore, it is always best to consult with a healthcare professional before using any herbal remedies for ED. Some herbs may also have interactions with other medications you are taking, or they may not be safe to use in certain situations, such as if you have high blood pressure or heart disease.

In conclusion, herbal remedies have been traditionally used to treat erectile dysfunction (ED) and some have been found to be effective in some men with ED. However, it's important to note that more research is needed to confirm these findings.

It's also important to talk to a healthcare professional before using any herbal remedies for ED, as some may have side effects or interact with other medications you are taking. Herbal remedies are not a substitute for professional medical advice, diagnosis, or treatment. Always seek the advice of a healthcare professional before starting any new treatment or discontinuing an existing treatment.

Herbs for prostate health

The prostate is a small gland located near the bladder in men that plays a role in sexual function and urine control. Prostate problems such as benign prostatic hyperplasia (BPH) and prostate cancer are common in men as they age. Herbal remedies have been traditionally used to improve prostate health and some have been found to be effective.

One herb that is commonly used for prostate health is saw palmetto. Saw palmetto is believed to work by blocking the production of dihydrotestosterone (DHT), a hormone that can contribute to the growth of the prostate. Studies have found that saw palmetto can help to reduce symptoms of BPH such as difficulty urinating and frequent urination. It is available in various forms such as capsules, teas, and topical solutions.

Another herb that is commonly used for prostate health is pygeum. Pygeum is an extract from the bark of the African plum tree, and it is believed to help reduce symptoms of BPH by reducing inflammation in the prostate. Studies have found that pygeum can help to reduce symptoms of BPH such as difficulty urinating and frequent urination. It is available in various forms such as capsules and teas.

Stinging Nettle is an herb that is commonly used for prostate health. It is believed to help reduce symptoms of BPH by reducing inflammation in the prostate. Studies have found that stinging nettle can help to reduce symptoms of BPH such as difficulty urinating and frequent urination. It is available in various forms such as capsules and teas.

Red Clover is an herb that is commonly used for prostate health. It is believed to help reduce symptoms of BPH by reducing inflammation in the prostate. Studies have found that red clover can help to reduce symptoms of BPH such as difficulty urinating and frequent urination. It is available in various forms such as capsules and teas.

It's important to note that while these herbs may be effective, they can also have side effects and may interact with other medications you are taking. Therefore, it is always best to consult with a healthcare professional before using any herbal remedies for prostate health. Some herbs may also have interactions with other medications you are taking, or they may not be safe to use in certain situations, such as if you are pregnant or breastfeeding.

In Conclusion, herbal remedies can be effective in improving prostate health, and saw palmetto, pygeum, stinging nettle, and red clover are some examples of herbs that are commonly used. However, it's important to note that more research is needed to confirm the effectiveness of these herbs and it's also important to talk to a healthcare professional before using any herbal remedies for prostate health, as some may have side effects or interact with other medications you are taking.

Herbal remedies are not a substitute for professional medical advice, diagnosis, or treatment. Always seek the advice of a healthcare professional before starting any new treatment or discontinuing an existing treatment. It's also important to note that these herbs are mostly used to improve the symptoms of benign prostatic hyperplasia (BPH) and not to treat or prevent prostate cancer. Therefore, it's always recommended to get regular check-ups and screenings with a healthcare professional to monitor any changes in prostate health.

Herbs for testosterone levels

Testosterone is a hormone that plays a vital role in the development of male characteristics and sexual function. Low testosterone levels can lead to a variety of symptoms such as decreased libido, erectile dysfunction, fatigue, and muscle loss. Herbal remedies have been traditionally used to increase testosterone levels, but it's important to note that more research is needed to confirm their effectiveness.

One herb that is commonly used to increase testosterone levels is Tribulus terrestris. Tribulus terrestris is a plant that is native to Europe, Asia and Africa. It is believed to increase the production of luteinizing hormone (LH), which in turn stimulates the production of testosterone. Studies have found that tribulus terrestris can help to improve sexual function and increase muscle mass, but more research is needed to confirm these findings.

Another herb that is commonly used to increase testosterone levels is ashwagandha. Ashwagandha is an adaptogen, which means it helps the body to better cope with stress. Studies have found that ashwagandha can help to increase testosterone levels and improve sperm quality.

Fenugreek is another herb that is commonly used to increase testosterone levels. Fenugreek is believed to increase the production of testosterone by stimulating the production of luteinizing hormone (LH). Studies have found that fenugreek can help to improve sexual function and increase muscle mass, but more research is needed to confirm these findings.

Ginger is an herb that is commonly used to increase testosterone levels. Ginger is a natural anti-inflammatory and antioxidant that can help to improve blood flow and increase the production of testosterone.

It's important to note that while these herbs may be effective, they can also have side effects and may interact with other medications you are taking. Therefore, it is always best to consult with a healthcare professional before using any herbal remedies for testosterone levels. Some herbs may also have interactions with other medications you are taking, or they may not be safe to use in certain situations, such as if you are pregnant or breastfeeding.

In conclusion, herbal remedies can be used to increase testosterone levels, and Tribulus terrestris, ashwagandha, fenugreek, and ginger are some examples of herbs that are commonly used. However, it's important to note that more research is needed to confirm the effectiveness of these herbs and it's also important to talk to a healthcare professional before using any herbal remedies for testosterone levels, as some may have side effects or interact with other medications you are taking. Herbal remedies are not a substitute for professional medical advice, diagnosis, or treatment. Always seek the advice of a healthcare professional before starting any new treatment or discontinuing an existing treatment.

Herbs for hair loss

Hair loss, also known as alopecia, is a common condition that can be caused by a variety of factors such as genetics, hormonal imbalances, medical conditions, and certain medications. Herbal remedies have been traditionally used to treat hair loss, and some have been found to be effective.

One herb that is commonly used for hair loss is saw palmetto. Saw palmetto is believed to work by blocking the production of dihydrotestosterone (DHT), which is a hormone that can contribute to hair loss. Studies have found that saw palmetto can help to reduce hair loss and improve hair growth. It is available in various forms such as capsules, teas, and topical solutions.

Another herb that is commonly used for hair loss is green tea. Green tea is a natural antioxidant that is believed to help improve hair growth by increasing blood flow to the scalp. Studies have found that green tea can help to reduce hair loss and improve hair growth. It is available in various forms such as tea, capsules, and topical solutions.

Ginseng is an herb that is commonly used for hair loss. It is believed to work by increasing blood flow to the scalp and promoting hair growth. Studies have found that ginseng can help to reduce hair loss and improve hair growth. It is available in various forms such as capsules, teas, and topical solutions.

Rosemary is an herb that is commonly used for hair loss. It is believed to work by increasing blood flow to the scalp and promoting hair growth. Studies have found that rosemary can help to reduce hair loss and improve hair growth. It is available in various forms such as essential oil, teas, and topical solutions.

It's important to note that while these herbs may be effective, they can also have side effects and may interact with other medications you are taking. Therefore, it is always best to consult with a healthcare professional before using any herbal remedies for hair loss. Some herbs may also have interactions with other medications you are taking, or they may not be safe to use in certain situations, such as if you are pregnant or breastfeeding.

In conclusion, herbal remedies can be effective in treating hair loss, and saw palmetto, green tea, ginseng, and rosemary are some examples of herbs that are commonly used. However, it's important to note that more research is needed to confirm the effectiveness of these herbs and it's also important to talk to a healthcare professional before using any herbal remedies for hair loss, as some may have side effects or interact with other medications you are taking. Herbal remedies are not a substitute for professional medical advice, diagnosis, or treatment. Always seek the advice of a healthcare professional before starting any new treatment or discontinuing an existing treatment.

Herbs for stress and anxiety

Stress and anxiety are common mental health conditions that can be caused by a variety of factors such as work, relationships, and financial issues. Herbal remedies have been traditionally used to treat stress and anxiety, and some have been found to be effective.

One herb that is commonly used for stress and anxiety is ashwagandha. Ashwagandha is an adaptogen, which means it helps the body to better cope with stress. Studies have found that ashwagandha can help to reduce stress and anxiety, as well as improve mood. It is available in various forms such as capsules, powders, and teas.

Another herb that is commonly used for stress and anxiety is passionflower. Passionflower is believed to work by increasing the levels of a chemical called GABA in the brain. GABA is a neurotransmitter that helps to reduce anxiety and promote relaxation. Passionflower is available in various forms such as capsules, teas, and tinctures.

Valerian is an herb that is commonly used as a natural sleep aid. It is also believed to help reduce anxiety and promote relaxation. Studies have found that valerian can help to reduce symptoms of anxiety, as well as improve sleep quality. It is available in various forms such as capsules, teas, and tinctures.

Lemon balm is an herb that is commonly used for anxiety and stress. It is believed to work by increasing the levels of GABA in the brain. Lemon balm is available in various forms such as capsules, teas, and tinctures.

Skullcap is an herb that is commonly used for anxiety, stress, and insomnia. It is believed to work by increasing the levels of GABA in the brain. Skullcap is available in various forms such as capsules, teas, and tinctures.

It's important to note that while these herbs may be effective, they can also have side effects and may interact with other medications you are taking. Therefore, it is always best to consult with a healthcare professional before using any herbal remedies for stress and anxiety. Some herbs may also have interactions with other medications you are taking, or they may not be safe to use in certain situations, such as if you are pregnant or breastfeeding.

In conclusion, herbal remedies can be effective in treating stress and anxiety, and ashwagandha, passionflower, valerian, lemon balm, and skullcap are some examples of herbs that are commonly used. However, it's important to note that more research is needed to confirm the effectiveness of these herbs and it's also important to talk to a healthcare professional before using any herbal remedies for stress and anxiety, as some may have side effects or interact with other medications you are taking. Herbal remedies are not a substitute for professional medical advice, diagnosis, or treatment. Always seek the advice of a healthcare professional before starting any new treatment or discontinuing an existing treatment.

Herbs For Digestion

Digestive problems can be caused by a variety of factors such as poor diet, stress, and certain medical conditions. Herbal remedies have been traditionally used to treat digestive problems, and some have been found to be effective. One such herb that is commonly used for digestive problems is senna.

Senna is a plant that is native to North Africa and has been used for centuries as a natural laxative. Senna contains compounds called sennosides, which stimulate the muscles in the walls of the colon, resulting in a bowel movement. It is particularly effective in treating constipation, and it is available in various forms such as tea, capsules, and tablets.

Senna can be used to relieve constipation, as well as to prepare the bowel for certain medical procedures such as colonoscopy. It is also used to relieve symptoms of hemorrhoids and to treat diverticulosis. It is also used as a weight loss aid, as it is believed that senna can help to reduce the absorption of fat and promote weight loss.

Senna is considered safe when used as directed and for short-term use. However, long-term use of senna can lead to a dependency on the herb, and it can also cause electrolyte imbalances, which can lead to muscle weakness, cramps, and irregular heartbeat. It should not be used by pregnant or breastfeeding women, or by children under the age of 12.

Other herbs that are commonly used for digestive problems include:

- Peppermint: Peppermint is a natural antispasmodic, which means it helps to relax the muscles in the gut and relieve cramping. Peppermint is also believed to help relieve symptoms of bloating and gas. Peppermint oil is commonly used to treat Irritable Bowel Syndrome (IBS) and other digestive problems.
- Ginger: Ginger is a natural anti-inflammatory and antioxidant that can help to relieve symptoms of indigestion, bloating, and gas. It is also believed to help relieve nausea and vomiting.
- Turmeric: Turmeric is a natural anti-inflammatory that can help to relieve symptoms of indigestion and bloating. It is also believed to help relieve symptoms of IBS.
- Fennel: Fennel is a natural antispasmodic that can help to relieve cramping, bloating, and gas. It is also believed to help relieve symptoms of IBS.
- Slippery Elm: Slippery Elm is a natural demulcent that can help to soothe the lining of the gut and relieve symptoms of indigestion and heartburn.

It's important to note that while these herbs may be effective, they can also have side effects and may interact with other medications you are taking. Therefore, it is always best to consult with a healthcare professional before using any herbal remedies for digestive problems. Some herbs may also have interactions with other medications you are taking, or they may not be safe to use in certain situations, such as if you are pregnant or breastfeeding.

In conclusion, herbal remedies can be effective in treating digestive problems, and senna is one such herb that is commonly used for constipation. However, it's important to note that more research is needed to confirm the effectiveness of these herbs and it's also important to talk to a healthcare professional before using any herbal remedies for digestive problems, as some may have side effects or interact with other medications you are taking. Herbal remedies are not a substitute for professional medical advice, diagnosis, or treatment. Always seek the advice of a healthcare professional before starting any new treatment or discontinuing an existing treatment.

How to prepare and use herbal remedies

There are several ways that men can prepare and use herbal remedies:

- Herbal teas: Herbal teas are a simple and convenient way to use herbs. To prepare an herbal tea, simply add the desired amount of dried herb (or a tea bag) to a cup of boiling water and allow it to steep for 5-10 minutes. Strain the herbs before drinking.
- Tinctures: Tinctures are liquid extracts made from herbs that are mixed with alcohol or glycerin. They are usually taken by dropperfuls, and the dosage can be adjusted to suit the individual needs. Tinctures can be used for internal and external use.
- Capsules: Capsules are a convenient way to take herbs. They are easy to swallow and can be taken with or without food. Capsules can be purchased pre-made or you can make your own by filling empty capsules with powdered herbs.
- Topical Applications: Some herbs can be used topically as ointments, creams, or oils. These remedies are applied to the skin for localized treatment of skin conditions, such as eczema, or for pain relief.
- Essential oils: Essential oils are concentrated plant extracts that can be used for aromatherapy, massage, or added to a

bath. They are usually used topically and should be diluted with a carrier oil before applying to the skin.

It's important to note that while herbal remedies can be effective, they can also have side effects and may interact with other medications you are taking. Therefore, it is always best to consult with a healthcare professional before using any herbal remedies. Some herbs may also have interactions with other medications you are taking, or they may not be safe to use in certain situations, such as if you are pregnant or breastfeeding.

It is also important to use high-quality herbs from reputable sources, to ensure that you are getting a pure and potent product. Keep in mind that some herbs can have negative interactions with certain prescription medications, so it's essential to check with your doctor before taking any herbal supplements.

In conclusion, herbal remedies can be a safe and effective way to treat a variety of health conditions, but it's essential to use them under the guidance of a healthcare professional and to use high-quality herbs from reputable sources.

Dosage recommendations

Herbal dosage recommendations can vary depending on the herb, the condition being treated, and the individual. In general, it's important to follow the dosage instructions on the product label or as recommended by a healthcare professional.

Here are some general guidelines for herbal dosage for men:

- Saw palmetto: 320-640 mg daily, standardized to contain 85-95% fatty acids and phytosterols
- Ashwagandha: 300-500 mg daily
- Fenugreek: 500-600 mg daily
- Ginger: 2-4g daily
- Tribulus terrestris: 250-750 mg daily
- Pygeum: 25-50 mg daily
- Stinging Nettle: 300-500 mg daily
- Red Clover: 2-4g daily
- Ginkgo Biloba: 120-240 mg daily, standardized to contain 24% flavone glycosides and 6% terpene lactones
- Horny Goat Weed (Epimedium): 100-200 mg daily, standardized to contain 10% icariin
- Maca: 1.5-3g daily
- Panax Ginseng: 200-400 mg daily, standardized to contain 4% ginsenosides

- Saw Palmetto: 320-640 mg daily, standardized to contain 85-95% fatty acids and phytosterols
- Tongkat Ali: 200-400 mg daily
- Turmeric: 500-2000 mg daily, standardized to contain 95% curcuminoids
- Black Cohosh: 40-80 mg daily, standardized to contain 2.5% triterpene glycosides
- Cranberry: 300-500 mg daily, standardized to contain 36-38% proanthocyanidins
- Echinacea: 4-8g per day of dried root or aerial parts
- Milk Thistle: 140-420 mg daily, standardized to contain 80-85% silymarin
- Saw palmetto: 320-640 mg daily, standardized to contain 85-95% fatty acids and phytosterols
- Turmeric: 400-600 mg of curcuminoids three times per day
- Valerian: 300-600mg of dried root or up to 1g of dried root for a liquid extract
- White willow bark: 240-320 mg daily, standardized to contain 15% salicin
- Yohimbe: 5-20 mg of yohimbine per day
- Zinc: 30-40mg per day

It's important to note that these are general guidelines and the recommended dosage may vary depending on the specific product or preparation. It's always best to consult with a healthcare professional before using any herbal remedies, as some may have side effects or interact with other medications you are taking.

It's also important to note that these recommendations are for short term use and long-term use should be discussed with a healthcare professional, as some herbs can have negative interactions with certain prescription medications, or they may not be safe to use in certain situations such as if you are pregnant or breastfeeding.

In conclusion, herbal dosage recommendations can vary depending on the herb, the condition being treated, and the individual. It's important to follow the dosage instructions on the product label or as recommended by a healthcare professional and to consult with a healthcare professional before using any herbal remedies, as some may have side effects or interact with other medications you are taking.

Potential side effects and interactions

While herbal remedies are generally considered to be safe
when used as directed, it is important to be aware of potential
side effects and interactions. Some herbs may interact with
other medications or have side effects of their own, so it is
important to speak with a healthcare professional before
taking any herbal remedy.

One of the most common side effects of herbal remedies is
an allergic reaction. Some people may be allergic to certain
herbs, and symptoms can include rash, hives, and difficulty
breathing. If you experience any of these symptoms, stop
taking the herb and seek medical attention immediately.

Some herbs can also interact with certain medications, and
this can be dangerous. For example, herbs like Ginkgo Biloba
can thin the blood, so they should not be taken with blood
thinning medications such as warfarin. Similarly, herbs like
Saw Palmetto can interfere with the absorption of certain
medications, so it is important to take them at least two hours
apart from other medications.

Some herbs can also have negative effects on certain
medical conditions. For example, herbs like Saw Palmetto
can increase the risk of bleeding in people with bleeding

disorders. Similarly, herbs like Ginkgo Biloba can increase the risk of seizures in people with a history of seizures.

Herbs can also have negative effects during pregnancy and breastfeeding, so it is important to speak with a healthcare professional before taking any herbal remedy if you are pregnant or breastfeeding.

It is also important to ensure that the herbs are obtained from a reputable source and are of high quality. Some herbs may be contaminated with other substances, such as heavy metals or pesticides, which can be dangerous. It is also important to ensure that the herbs are used in the appropriate dosage and preparation.

In conclusion, while herbal remedies can be an effective and safe alternative to traditional medications, it is important to be aware of potential side effects and interactions. Always consult a healthcare professional before taking any herbal remedy, and to ensure that the herbs are obtained from a reputable source. Be aware of the dosage and preparation, and pay attention to the symptoms you may have. Be extra cautious if you are pregnant, breastfeeding or have other medical conditions.

Storing and preserving herbal remedies

Proper storage and preservation of herbal remedies is important to ensure their effectiveness and safety. Here are some tips on how to store and preserve herbal remedies:

- Store herbal remedies in a cool, dry place, away from direct sunlight and heat. This will help to prevent the herbs from losing their potency and becoming rancid.
- Store herbal remedies in airtight containers, such as glass jars with tight-fitting lids. This will help to prevent the herbs from absorbing moisture and becoming moldy.
- Keep herbs away from strong odors, as they can absorb the smells, which can affect the quality and effectiveness of the herbs.
- Label the herbal remedies with the name of the herb, the date of purchase, and the expiration date. This will help to keep track of the freshness of the herbs and ensure that they are used before they expire.
- Dried herbs can be stored for up to a year, while tinctures and extracts can be stored for up to two years.
- Some herbs can be stored in the freezer, to help them last longer. However, keep in mind that freezing can affect the potency of the herbs, so it's best to consult with a healthcare professional before freezing any herbs.

- Keep in mind that some herbs may lose their potency over time, so it's important to use them within the recommended time frame.
- Avoid buying herbs in bulk, only purchase what you need for a short period of time.
- Do not store herbal remedies in plastic containers as they can react with the herbs and affect the quality.

In conclusion, proper storage and preservation of herbal remedies is important to ensure their effectiveness and safety. Herbal remedies should be stored in a cool, dry place, away from direct sunlight and heat. They should be stored in airtight containers, labeled with the name of the herb, the date of purchase, and the expiration date. Dried herbs can be stored for up to a year, while tinctures and extracts can be stored for up to two years. Some herbs can be stored in the freezer, but it's best to consult with a healthcare professional before freezing any herbs. Avoid buying herbs in bulk, and do not store herbal remedies in plastic containers

Conclusion

In conclusion, herbal remedies have been used for centuries to improve men's health and wellness. Herbs can be used to treat a wide range of issues such as prostate health, sexual dysfunction, stress, and anxiety. They can also help to support the liver, cardiovascular system, digestive system and more.

Herbal remedies are a natural alternative to traditional medications, and they can be used in the form of teas, tinctures, and capsules. They can also be used in conjunction with other treatments to provide additional benefits. Herbs are also known to have less side effects than traditional medications, making them a popular choice for many men.

It is important to remember that not all herbs may be suitable for everyone and it is important to consult a healthcare professional before taking any herbal remedy. Additionally, during pregnancy, breastfeeding or taking medications it is important to consult with a healthcare professional before taking any herbal remedy. This is to ensure that the herbs are compatible with other medications and that there are no adverse reactions.

It is also important to ensure that the herbs are obtained from a reputable source and that they are stored and preserved properly. Herbs should be kept in a cool, dry place, away from light and heat, to ensure that they retain their potency and effectiveness.

Herbal remedies can be a great way to improve men's health and wellness, but it's important to remember that they should be used with caution. By following these guidelines, men can use herbal remedies safely and effectively to improve their health and well-being.

Furthermore, it is important to note that herbal remedies should be used as a complement rather than a replacement for conventional medical treatment when needed. If a man is experiencing any symptoms that are severe or persistent, it is essential to consult with a healthcare professional.

In conclusion, herbal remedies can be a valuable addition to a men's health and wellness routine, but it's important to use them responsibly, with the guidance of a healthcare professional. With the right approach, men can harness the power of herbs to improve their health and well-being, while minimizing any potential risks.

It is important to remember that herbal remedies are not a quick fix, they should be used as a complement to a healthy lifestyle and regular check-ups with a healthcare professional.

By taking a holistic approach and utilizing the benefits of herbal remedies, men can achieve optimal health and vitality for a happier and healthier life.

Herbal remedies for men's health

Herbal remedies have been used for centuries to treat a wide range of health conditions, and they continue to be a popular alternative to traditional medications. Herbal remedies are made from natural ingredients, and they can be used to treat a variety of men's health issues, including prostate problems, sexual dysfunction, hair loss, stress and anxiety, infertility, and cardiovascular health.

One of the most common men's health issues that herbal remedies can help with is prostate problems. Herbs like Saw Palmetto have been found to be effective in treating symptoms of an enlarged prostate and may also have anti-cancer properties. Saw Palmetto works by blocking the conversion of testosterone to dihydrotestosterone (DHT), which can cause prostate enlargement.

Sexual dysfunction is another common men's health issue that herbal remedies can help with. Herbs like Horny Goat Weed, Tribulus Terrestris and Ginkgo Biloba have been found to be effective in improving sexual function and treating symptoms of erectile dysfunction. These herbs work by increasing blood flow to the penis and boosting levels of testosterone.

Hair loss and male pattern baldness are also common men's health issues that herbal remedies can help with. Herbs like Saw Palmetto and Ginkgo Biloba have been found to be effective in preventing hair loss and promoting hair growth. Saw Palmetto

Herbs For Cancer

There are a number of herbs that have been traditionally used to support cancer treatment, however, it is important to note that research on the effectiveness of these herbs is still limited and it is important to consult with a healthcare professional before taking any herbal remedy. Additionally, herbal remedies should not be used as a replacement for conventional medical treatment. Here are a few examples of herbs that have been used for cancer:

- Turmeric: Turmeric contains a compound called curcumin, which has been shown to have anti-inflammatory and antioxidant properties. Some studies have suggested that curcumin may have anti-cancer effects and may help to inhibit the growth of cancer cells.
- Milk Thistle: Milk thistle is known to have antioxidant and anti-inflammatory properties, and it may help to support liver function. The liver plays a key role in detoxifying the body and eliminating toxins, which can be beneficial for people undergoing cancer treatment.
- Echinacea: Echinacea has been traditionally used to support the immune system and may help to reduce the risk of infections in people undergoing cancer treatment.

- Saw Palmetto: Saw Palmetto is traditionally used to support prostate health, and it may help to reduce inflammation in the prostate gland.
- Black Cohosh: Black cohosh is traditionally used to support the health of the reproductive system, and it may help to reduce symptoms of menopause.
- Red Clover: Red clover is traditionally used to support the health of the bones, and it may help to reduce the risk of osteoporosis.
- Guggulu: Guggulu is traditionally used to support the health of the cardiovascular system, and it may help to reduce the risk of heart disease.
- Astragalus: Astragalus is traditionally used to support the immune system and may help to reduce the risk of infections in people undergoing cancer treatment.
- Reishi mushroom: Reishi mushroom is traditionally used to support the immune system, and it may help to reduce the risk of infections in people undergoing cancer Green Tea: Green tea contains a compound called EGCG (epigallocatechin-3-gallate), which has been shown to have antioxidant and anti-inflammatory properties. Some studies have suggested that EGCG may help to inhibit the growth of cancer cells, particularly in the colon, breast, lung, and prostate.
- Cat's Claw: Cat's claw is traditionally used to support the immune system and may help to reduce inflammation throughout the body. Some studies have suggested that it

may help to inhibit the growth of cancer cells, particularly in the stomach and intestinal tract.

- Black Pepper: Black pepper contains a compound called piperine, which has been shown to have antioxidant and anti-inflammatory properties. Some studies have suggested that piperine may help to inhibit the growth of cancer cells, particularly in the liver, stomach, and colon.
- Holy Basil: Holy basil is traditionally used to support the immune system and may help to reduce inflammation throughout the body. Some studies have suggested that it may help to inhibit the growth of cancer cells, particularly in the lung and skin.
- Ginger: Ginger contains compounds called gingerols and shogaols, which have been shown to have anti-inflammatory and antioxidant properties. Some studies have suggested that ginger may help to inhibit the growth of cancer cells, particularly in the colon, prostate, and ovarian. Treatment.
- Dandelion: Dandelion is known to have diuretic properties, and it may help to support the health of the kidneys and liver.
- Burdock: Burdock is known to have blood purifying properties, and it may help to support the health of the liver and skin.
- Nettle: Nettle is known to have anti-inflammatory properties, and it may help to support the health of the joints and respiratory system.

- Yellow dock: Yellow dock is known to have blood purifying properties, and it may help to support the health of the liver and skin.
- Astragalus: Astragalus is traditionally used to support the immune system and may help to reduce the risk of infections in people undergoing cancer treatment.
- Aloe vera: Aloe vera is traditionally used to support the health of the skin, and it may help to reduce inflammation and promote healing.
- Kelp: Kelp is known to have anti-inflammatory properties, and it may help to support the health of the thyroid and metabolism.
- Lemon grass: Lemongrass is known to have anti-inflammatory properties, and it may help to support the health of the digestive system and reduce stress.
- Marshmallow: Marshmallow is known to have anti-inflammatory properties, and it may help to support the health of the digestive system and respiratory system.
- Chlorophyll-rich herbs such as wheatgrass, barley grass, spirulina, alfalfa and chlorella are considered alkaline herbs, they can help to balance the pH levels of the body and neutralize acidity.
- Holy basil: Holy basil is known to have adaptogenic properties, which means it can help the body adapt to stress. It may also support the health of the adrenal glands, which play a key role in regulating the body's stress response.

- Ginkgo biloba: Ginkgo biloba is known to have antioxidant properties and may help to support the health of the brain and improve circulation.
- Licorice root: Licorice root is known to have anti-inflammatory properties and may help to support the health of the digestive system and the respiratory system.
- Milk thistle: Milk thistle is known to have antioxidant properties and may help to support the health of the liver, it also helps detoxifying the body and eliminating toxins.
- Saw palmetto: Saw palmetto is traditionally used to support the health of the prostate and urinary tract.
- Echinacea: Echinacea is traditionally used to support the immune system and may help to reduce the risk of infections in people undergoing cancer treatment.
- Black cohosh: Black cohosh is traditionally used to support the health of the reproductive system, and it may help to reduce symptoms of menopause.
- Red clover: Red clover is traditionally used to support the health of the bones, and it may help to reduce the risk of osteoporosis.
- Guggulu: Guggulu is traditionally used to support the health of the cardiovascular system, and it may help to reduce the risk of heart disease.
- Burdock root : is traditionally used to support the health of the liver, skin and blood.

- Saw Palmetto - Prostate health
- Ginkgo Biloba - Cardiovascular health
- Tribulus Terrestris - Sexual dysfunction and infertility
- Ashwagandha - Stress and anxiety
- Horny Goat Weed - Sexual dysfunction
- Maca Root - Infertility
- Epimedium - Sexual dysfunction
- Panax Ginseng - Cardiovascular health and energy levels
- Cordyceps Sinensis - Cardiovascular health and energy levels
- Turmeric - Anti-inflammatory and joint health
- Ginger - Anti-inflammatory and digestive health
- Milk Thistle - Liver health and detoxification
- Dandelion - Liver health and detoxification
- Bacopa Monnieri - Cognitive function and memory
- St. John's Wort - Anxiety and depression
- Passionflower - Anxiety and depression
- Echinacea - Immune system health
- Goldenseal - Immune system health
- Peppermint - Digestive health
- Fennel - Digestive health

1. Saw Palmetto tea - To make this tea, steep 1 teaspoon of dried Saw Palmetto berries in a cup of hot water for 10 minutes. Drink 1-2 cups a day to help with prostate health.

2. Ginkgo Biloba tea - To make this tea, steep 1 teaspoon of dried Ginkgo Biloba leaves in a cup of hot water for 10 minutes. Drink 1-2 cups a day to help with cardiovascular health and sexual dysfunction.

3. Horny Goat Weed tea - To make this tea, steep 1 teaspoon of dried Horny Goat Weed in a cup of hot water for 10 minutes. Drink 1-2 cups a day to help with sexual dysfunction.

4. Tribulus Terrestris tea - To make this tea, steep 1 teaspoon of dried Tribulus Terrestris in a cup of hot water for 10 minutes. Drink 1-2 cups a day to help with sexual dysfunction and infertility.

5. Ashwagandha tea - To make this tea, steep 1 teaspoon of dried Ashwagandha root in a cup of hot water for 10 minutes. Drink 1-2 cups a day to help with stress and anxiety.

6. Milk Thistle tea - To make this tea, steep 1 teaspoon of dried Milk Thistle seeds in a cup of hot water for 10 minutes. Drink 1-2 cups a day to help with liver health and detoxification.

7. Turmeric tea - To make this tea, steep 1 teaspoon of turmeric powder in a cup of hot water for 10 minutes. Drink

1-2 cups a day to help with anti-inflammatory and joint health.

8. Maca Root tea - To make this tea, steep 1 teaspoon of dried Maca Root powder in a cup of hot water for 10 minutes. Drink 1-2 cups a day to help with hormonal balance and energy levels.

9. Cordyceps Sinensis tea - To make this tea, steep 1 teaspoon of dried Cordyceps Sinensis in a cup of hot water for 10 minutes. Drink 1-2 cups a day to help with cardiovascular health and energy levels.

10. Saw Palmetto Tincture - To make this tincture, mix 1:5 ratio of Saw Palmetto berries and alcohol (such as vodka) in a glass jar. Shake well and let it sit for 2 weeks in a dark place. Take 1-2 droppers full a day to help with prostate health and hair loss.

11. Dandelion Root tea - To make this tea, steep 1 teaspoon of dried Dandelion Root in a cup of hot water for 10 minutes. Drink 1-2 cups a day to help with liver health and detoxification.

12. Echinacea tea - To make this tea, steep 1 teaspoon of dried Echinacea in a cup of hot water for 10 minutes. Drink 1-2 cups a day to help with immune system health.

13. Panax Ginseng tea - To make this tea, steep 1 teaspoon of dried Panax Ginseng in a cup of hot water for 10 minutes. Drink 1-2 cups a day to help with cardiovascular health and energy levels.

14. Saw Palmetto Tincture - To make this tincture, mix 1:5 ratio of Saw Palmetto berries and alcohol (such as vodka) in a glass jar. Shake well and let it sit for 2 weeks in a dark place. Take 1-2 droppers full a day to help with prostate health and hair loss.

15. Horny Goat Weed Tincture - To make this tincture, mix 1:5 ratio of Horny Goat Weed and alcohol (such as vodka) in a glass jar. Shake well and let it sit for 2 weeks in a dark place. Take 1-2 droppers full a day to help with sexual dysfunction.

16. Tribulus Terrestris Tincture - To make this tincture, mix 1:5 ratio of Tribulus Terrestris and alcohol (such as vodka) in a glass jar. Shake well and let it sit for 2 weeks in a dark place. Take 1-2 droppers full a day to help with sexual dysfunction and infertility.

17. Maca Root Tincture - To make this tincture, mix 1:5 ratio of Maca Root powder and alcohol (such as vodka) in a glass jar. Shake well and let it sit for 2 weeks in a dark place. Take 1-2 droppers full a day to help with hormonal balance and energy levels.

18. Cordyceps Sinensis Tincture - To make this tincture, mix 1:5 ratio of Cordyceps Sinensis and alcohol (such as vodka) in a glass jar. Shake well and let it sit for 2 weeks in a dark place. Take 1-2 droppers full a day to help with cardiovascular health and energy levels.

19. Saw Palmetto/Nettle Root Tincture - To make this tincture, mix 1:5 ratio of Saw Palmetto berries and nettle root in

alcohol (such as vodka) in a glass jar. Shake well and let it sit for 2 weeks in a dark place. Take 1-2 droppers full a day to help with prostate health and hair loss.

20. Ginkgo Biloba Tincture - To make this tincture, mix 1:5 ratio of Ginkgo Biloba and alcohol (such as vodka) in a glass jar. Shake well and let it sit for 2 weeks in a dark place. Take 1-2 droppers full a day to help with cardiovascular health and sexual dysfunction.

21. Milk Thistle Tincture - To make this tincture, mix 1:5 ratio of Milk Thistle seeds and alcohol (such as vodka) in a glass jar. Shake well and let it sit for 2 weeks in a dark place. Take 1-2 droppers full a day to help with liver health and detoxification.

22. Dandelion Root Tincture - To make this tincture, mix 1:5 ratio of Dandelion Root and alcohol (such as vodka) in a glass jar. Shake well and let it sit for 2 weeks in a dark place. Take 1-2 droppers full a day to help with liver health and detoxification.

23. Turmeric Tincture - To make this tincture, mix 1:5 ratio of Turmeric powder and alcohol (such as vodka) in a glass jar. Shake well and let it sit for 2 weeks in a dark place. Take 1-2 droppers full a day to help with anti-inflammatory and joint health.

24. Ashwagandha Tincture - To make this tincture, mix 1:5 ratio of Ashwagandha root and alcohol (such as vodka) in a glass jar. Shake well and let it sit for 2 weeks in a dark

place. Take 1-2 droppers full a day to help with stress and anxiety.

42. Panax Ginseng Tincture - To make this tincture, mix 1:5 ratio of Panax Ginseng and alcohol (such as vodka) in a glass jar. Shake well and let it sit for 2 weeks in a dark place. Take 1-2 droppers full a day to help with cardiovascular health and energy levels.

43. Saw Palmetto/Pygeum Tincture - To make this tincture, mix 1:5 ratio of Saw Palmetto berries and Pygeum in alcohol (such as vodka) in a glass jar. Shake well and let it sit for 2 weeks in a dark place. Take 1-2 droppers full a day to help with prostate health.

44. Saw Palmetto/Stinging Nettle Tincture - To make this tincture, mix 1:5 ratio of Saw Palmetto berries and Stinging Nettle in alcohol (such as vodka) in a glass jar. Shake well and let it sit for 2 weeks in a dark place. Take 1-2 droppers full a day to help with prostate health and hair loss.

45. Saw Palmetto/Zinc Tincture - To make this tincture, mix 1:5 ratio of Saw Palmetto berries, zinc and alcohol (such as vodka) in a glass jar. Shake well and let it sit for 2 weeks in a dark place. Take 1-2 droppers full a day to help with prostate health and male fertility.

Notes and Reflections:

Notes and Reflections

Notes and Reflections

www.ingramcontent.com/pod-product-compliance
Lightning Source LLC
Chambersburg PA
CBHW081603250726
48653CB00009B/3547